Growing Older Looking Younger

The Secrets To Looking Young And Staying Healthy For Men And Women

Dr. Jose Pearson

TABLE OF CONTENTS

CHAPTER 1
HOW WE AGE

No matter how old you become, your body was created to remain healthy, powerful, and pain-free for the whole of your life. Your body has the capacity to continuously mend itself after injury because of genetic programming. Your living machine's main goal is to repair, whether that means fixing damaged bones, torn muscles, wounds, and burns, or fending off invaders with its immune army cells. Additionally, the more you exercise, the more you encourage your body's remarkable cellular regeneration and beneficial, adaptive reactions to stress.

Yes, your body was designed with intricate mechanisms that can keep you healthy and active far into your later years. Your muscles, not your heart, brain, or lungs, are the sharpest, most potent, or most adaptable instrument for maintaining this bright freshness. Long after you reach old age, your muscles have a natural tendency to stay strong and flexible. a feature that not only makes you feel and move better but also enhances the performance of each and every bodily system.

Amazing turnarounds are conceivable for persons who start exercising late in life or who were previously entirely inactive. I've been in awe of people in their forties, fifties, sixties, and even seventies who enjoy their ability to run a road race, hike mountain trails, apply for (and get!) a difficult new promotion at work, or even just twirl their kids or grandchildren around in the air, all because they get just a little bit of exercise every day.

All of these folks share the knowledge that if you exercise, you'll never have to lose muscle mass and can maintain your youthful vigor, energy, power, and vitality permanently. And you may get the majority of these advantages with only 30 minutes of daily activity. I've worked with the ESSENTRICS method to teach thousands of individuals how to exercise in a way that is completely different from the harmful, ineffective "no pain, no gain" mentality of the past. In comparison, I'd argue the "no pain, all joy" school of exercise is eccentrics. In the time it takes you to watch one episode of television, you may use my program to strengthen your muscles, guard your body against chronic illness, acquire a ton of energy, and get to enjoy a long and slim "dancer's body" as a bonus.

Not to mention the main benefit: You'll live longer. In a recent longitudinal research, data from more than 650,000 individuals whose medical records had been kept for 10 years were reviewed. The researchers' astounding results included the fact that exercising increases life expectancy by 7 minutes for every minute spent exercising. These results were seen in individuals who began working out at the age of 45 and exercised for only 150 minutes a week, which is equivalent to doing the ESSENTRICS program five times a week and that was only the beginning.

People who exercised more often had much better outcomes. An incredible ratio of a guaranteed 1-to-7 return on your investment. That type of return is unbeatable in any stock market. Isn't it incredible?

For these types of health benefits, you don't need to be an athlete, a professional dancer, or a genetic lottery winner.

You just need to stretch for roughly 30 minutes a day using a very precise, scientifically proven method. But before we learn about the program itself, let's go a bit further to discover why the muscles are so crucial for maintaining and improving the health of every system, as well as how we may immediately make use of their diverse abilities. I thought that chronological years were what determined the loss of muscle mass and decline in vitality until I began learning about aging.

I've always believed that certain people's ability to remain young and energetic as they aged while others did not was a question of good fortune or excellent genes. In actuality, genes hardly even factor into it. According to research, only 25% of our lifespan is thought to be influenced by our genes; the remaining 75% is thought to be influenced by our way of life and our environment.

Exercise is another important component that may extend our lives by up to 8 years, making it one of the most important ones overall. Through the wonder of a daily dosage of gentle stretching exercise, all of our bodily systems including our bones, heart, and even skin can remain healthy and strong for the remainder of our lives.

This fundamental reality has not always been known to us. Many of us have had a close call with mortality at some point in our lives, either as a result of a terrible accident or a condition like cancer or heart disease. We considered frail bones, hunched posture, and staggering gait to be normal signs of aging. Yes, such symptoms may be considered "normal" and "natural"; what we saw was the body's typical deconditioning and muscular degradation process. However, just because a process occurs naturally does not imply it is inescapable.

Think about the alternatives available to each gardener: Her plants will thrive and expand if she takes good care of her garden, meticulously watering it, and making sure it receives the proper amount of sunlight, nutrients, and water. But if she doesn't take care of her garden, it will soon be overrun with weeds, and the plants won't have enough food or water to survive. These two results are equally "natural."

These are two options with two distinct outcomes that both abide by the rules of nature. But nobody would contest that they both deserve to be happy. Due to a lack of knowledge, many individuals used to allow their bodies to age prematurely. Do you recall how unusual it once seemed to encounter an old person with excellent posture and vigor, a senior who lived without chronic pain or any health issues, roughly twenty years ago?

Those individuals were regarded as exceptional and remarkable in the not-too-distant past. Today, we encounter a lot of individuals who are radiantly healthy at 60, 70, 80, and even 90 years old. We see professors doing scientific research into their nineties, 93-year-old yoga instructors, and presidents of state who continue to rule into their late eighties. At 92 years old, Betty White is still making people laugh and entertaining crowds. We are just now beginning to realize how much control we have over good aging. So what does eternal vitality entail? Many individuals ponder how their lives could change if they made the time commitment necessary to follow the eccentric's program. You may live your whole life with great posture, I assure them. The body is built to have and work with excellent posture, thus it is more natural to have great posture than to have a slouched back.

Slouching is brought on by the musculature's breakdown from lack of usage. Slouching is the human counterpart of a plant getting strangled by the weeds around it, resulting in the premature death of the muscle cells. However, the most natural and healthful position for the spine is one with excellent posture. The torso's muscles are designed to be powerful and adaptable. The health of our spinal muscles will keep our posture upright and improve the efficiency of all of our internal organs. The body is built to walk with a spring in its stride. A light, relaxed gait may be readily powered by the muscles of the feet, ankles, knees, and hips, which are designed to be powerful enough to do so. Even a little exercise will maintain those muscles strong and flexible. Neglect causes those muscles to shrivel and atrophy.

You will feel youthful even as you age if you do walk with this sort of lightness and agility. You will also be less likely to have any aches, pains, or stiffness. The majority of aches and pains are caused by atrophied, inflexible muscles, and if they are not addressed, they will only become worse as we age. In actuality, the majority of chronic aches and pains associated with the muscles are completely unnecessary. Our muscles will give us a spring in our step that lasts the rest of our lives if we train them with equal focus on strength and flexibility.

Uncontrollable weight gain may seem to be an inevitable part of getting older, but it may be completely avoided by doing the right strengthening and flexibility activities. Weak, rigid muscles make us seem floppy and formless, and those unneeded physical alterations deprive us of our confidence and self-worth. Indeed, we may not always be sprinting down the beach in bikinis. Yet who really wants that?

Through frequent easy full-body stretching and strengthening exercises, we can easily maintain a trim waist and narrow hips, even develop muscle definition and drastically decrease the dreaded "softening" in our midsections. I think I've made my point now. Since we now know it may be prevented, the fast deterioration of the human body is not an inevitable process that must be accepted and suffered. But for many of us, the concern is: How can we stop it from happening? What are the next steps?

Even if you follow a regular workout schedule, chronic pain may cause frequent interruptions in your routine. Or maybe you are losing weight via food but are unsure of the kind of exercise you need to be performing. Or you could have put all of your efforts into a challenging workout regimen only to become frustrated, burn out, and develop a bad habit of inactivity while waiting for the next item to motivate you.

Simply stated, a lot of folks are in a rut and have no idea where to start. How do we get started? We may watch the marathon runners or the spin class addicts and realize that's not for us. Is it more crucial to concentrate on cardio or strength training? Should we exercise at a low level for a long period of time or at a high intensity for a short period of time? A program may be delayed to a less hectic period. Debating one software that would be superior to another might take some time. Which one of them do I do? may cross our minds as we peruse the workout equipment or book section.

Every time I overhear someone asking these questions, I am eager to introduce them to ESSENTRICS. Because I am certain that individuals can achieve a wide range of health and fitness objectives with this one program. The same routine works for everyone, regardless of whether you're currently in excellent condition, are just starting back into fitness, or have never been active in your life. Here's why:

- You can perform it anyplace, whether indoors or outdoors; as long as there is one body length of space available.

- No equipment is required. You don't even need nice shoes to work out in your jammies. (ESSENTRICS should be performed barefoot!)

- Time is not a big factor. The whole workout may be finished in about 30 minutes.

- You don't have to be really fit. The ESSENTRICS program progresses, beginning off easy and increasing in difficulty as you go.

- You'll never experience "pain." The ESSENTRICS program is soothing and focuses on getting all of your muscles loose and flexible as you strengthen them.

- Losing weight is possible without perspiring. One incredible quality of ESSENTRICS is how well it can shape your body, assisting you in building stronger muscles that burn fat as you sleep.

All you need is a little assistance from this daily simple full-body workout to feel young and healthy. Because we've been taught that exercise must hurt and that we must push ourselves to the limit in order to see benefits, you may be astonished to learn that something so mild can be so helpful. But a lot of individuals dread doing intense exercise. The fact is that we don't have to strain our bodies beyond their breaking point in order to stay flexible and strong.

Even a little amount of exercise will have an exponential value return. If you have never liked the notion of exercising, you have definitely attempted some difficult, strange, and draining routines. The ESSENTRICS program will demonstrate how 30 minutes of exercise may be enjoyable and enjoyable, which is how exercising should really feel natural. You'll rediscover the thrill of exercise and begin to anticipate your subsequent workouts. If you're a seasoned exerciser, you'll be amazed and ecstatic to learn about stretching, strengthening, lengthening, and toning technique that leaves you feeling so calm and limber and that also produces such great benefits in only 30 minutes a day. I think ESSENTRICS will fundamentally alter how you see physical activity.

The concept for the ESSENTRICS model first came to me as a young girl when I was a student at the National Ballet School of Canada and later while I was performing professionally with the National Ballet Company. There, I honed a discipline and inventiveness that stimulated my mind for inquiry and discovery, although I wouldn't master the skills until much later. I also gained a deep understanding of form and body. I first had to comprehend the requirement.

I quit the firm and began my own business after dancing in far too many Nutcracker productions, but I was eventually drawn back into the corporate world. I loved the glitzy but exhausting travel schedule that required me to leave my 5-year-old daughter with family for two weeks each month. Even though at the time it looked the most reckless, quitting that job was the finest choice I've ever made.

I was unemployed and unsure about how I would support my daughter Sahra on my own. To make ends meet, I began instructing fitness courses at a nearby church. My aerobics lessons quickly became well-known thanks to positive word of mouth, and before I knew it, I was instructing almost five sessions a day in the basement of a church. I realized I was outgrowing the space and made the bold decision to start my own training facility.

As I spoke about my research with more and more individuals, both within and outside the fitness industry, I came to the conclusion that most people didn't really like working out. The students at my studio appreciated my sessions, no doubt, but over time I started to notice how many individuals were passing by my door without ever setting foot inside and exercising. It captivated me. Why did they not appreciate what brought me such delight and satisfaction? I polled a large number of individuals who didn't exercise to discover, and what I learned was that people truly wanted to exercise but they simply didn't like the options available.

Although aerobics had revolutionized the fitness industry, there were many criticisms of it as well. Many people were deterred from participating by the loud music, impactful motions, profuse perspiration, and bulky muscular tone they seemed to acquire. I often heard from my clients, particularly the ladies, that they preferred fluid exercises that stretched them out rather than made them bulky. I want a long, lean, and slim physique. In other words, the physique of a dancer.

I'm sure I could be of assistance with it! I set out to develop an "anti-aerobic" exercise regimen. I delved deeply into the fields of anatomy, physiology, and fundamental kinesiology with the help of extensive study and the essential guidance of Dr. Shibata, head of oncology and surgery at Montreal's Royal Victoria Hospital, and Fiona Gilmore, a former sports physiotherapist. I had the opportunity to provide trial sessions to a select number of students as the center's owner, and they helped me develop a program that was enjoyable, therapeutic, and, most importantly, helped them slim down and tone their bodies the way they had thought exercise would.

The core of the ESSENTRICS technique, which I refer to as the Esmonde Technique and which serves as the basis for this book and all the other fitness regimens I have ever created, was born out of these courses. All of these courses were designed to keep students active and healthy from birth to death. My first lesson was called Ancient Stretch because the exercises stretched the muscles in the manner of classical architecture, with long, slender, graceful lines.

The moment I started offering public Classical Stretch lessons at my gym, they were quite popular.

They were so well-liked that I had to teach additional teachers my method in order to meet the demand. The need to train others compelled me to put my approach down on paper so that it might be taught to others. Before I could teach anybody else the method, I had to analyze it and determine what it was. I read every book on anatomy, physiology, and medicine I could get my hands on at that period.

This was the start of a 10-year process in which I wrote my own manuals, tested them, and then started again. Before finishing a set of four manuals, levels one through four, the foundation of our teacher-training program, I went through that procedure three times. When the program unexpectedly saw such rapid development in 1999, I summoned the confidence to contact PBS in the vain hope that it could be open to running my fitness show on their network. The rest is history, I suppose.

Millions of American homes still have access to Classical Stretch everyday fifteen years after its debut. Numerous Americans get out of bed every day to participate in the program. In order to effectively teach individuals, we've worked throughout the years to provide better explanations for this potent technique. Many people have said that they see ESSENTRICS as a flexibility program that incorporates certain aspects of tai chi, some physiotherapy stretching, and a lengthening of the muscles akin to ballet. We were certain that our program, which we called Classical Stretch, was a flexibility program since everyone who participated in it improved their flexibility.

However, consider this: The TV show's viewers as well as our own customers continued to send us testimonies describing how their strength, weight, and body form had dramatically changed. If they persisted, people discovered that ESSENTRICS would lengthen their legs, hips, and stomach in addition to their arms, neck, and shoulders, improve their posture, slenderize their shoulders, lengthen their pectorals and upper back, open up their chests and elongate their necklines, reduce love handles, and get rid of underarm flab. They weren't the only ones seeing these effects after a few weeks of rigorous ESSENTRICS.

They discovered that using a measuring device and a camera allowed them to capture shocking changes in the size and structure of their muscles. Many dropped one or more pant sizes. We were perplexed. We didn't believe that stretching could be responsible for significant modifications in strength, weight, and body composition. Even though we were aware that participants in the program were losing weight, we were unable to determine why. We ultimately discovered the definition of Classical Stretch in the study of movement and muscle architecture.

We had a revelation. Sports science states that there are two methods to build your muscles: eccentrically or concentrically. While eccentric workouts extend the muscle, concentrated activities shorten the muscle, strengthening it. Concentric strengthening is the main emphasis of most other exercise regimens. In the gym, you can observe concentric strengthening every day when individuals tighten and shorten their quadriceps muscles while attempting to, for example, straighten a leg on a leg extension machine, pull a hand weight toward their shoulders while performing a biceps curl, or "crunch" their abdominal muscles while performing sit-ups.

Usually, we devote all of our training concentration to that concentric action and pay less attention to stretching our muscles. But by disregarding this, we're neglecting a crucial component of eccentric training that helps build healthy, powerful muscles. While equally important to concentric exercise in terms of lengthening and strengthening, eccentric exercise is often disregarded as "wasted" time. When you reach into a high cabinet or exit a moving vehicle, your body is really doing eccentric workouts.

For example, when you get up, you bend your knee and extend your quadriceps while they are still supporting the whole weight of your body. While extending, you are strengthening. Eccentric exercise enables your "lever" (muscle) to easily tolerate greater resistance when in its stretched position, similar to the physics axiom "The longer the lever, the heavier the load." Muscles that are both extended and stronger as a consequence.

When we recognized that the fundamental underlying Classical Stretch was eccentric exercise, we quickly understood why individuals were losing weight while following our program. Because muscle cells burn more calories, increasing the intensity of the load on the longer muscle results in an increase in muscle mass, an increase in metabolic rate, a greater caloric expenditure, and weight loss.

Along the way, we have seen several persons practicing ESSENTRICS or adhering to Classical Stretch who effortlessly dropped weight and inches in their alleged problem areas, lengthening and toning their bodies. All of this is possible using a technique that just requires 30 minutes every day. I'd want to show you a complete body makeover similar to this one.

CHAPTER 2
OUR PERCEPTION OF YOUTH

To fully comprehend good aging, one must start with the fundamental units of the body: the cells. Numerous billions of cells make up your body. Every tissue in your body exhibits the health and vitality of your cells. The health of your cells dictates how your body will react to each of these activities, regardless of whether you can run and jump, sing or laugh spontaneously, have a quiet day with friends, or stand on the dais in front of your peers to give a speech.

Your body will respond naturally with energy if your cells are properly fed and stimulated. You will also be able to handle stress, maintain a healthy blood pressure and blood sugar level, and maintain a young, bright appearance. Your cells begin to atrophy and die if they are not properly supplied and stimulated, which may cause you to feel lethargic, unhappy, and in pain. You could be inclined to dismiss the relevance of some cell death since you have billions of cells, after all. However, every single cell matters when it comes to Growing Older Looking Younger, thus you don't want to let any of them suffer any damage.

Brain cells, nerve cells, blood cells, hair cells, egg cells, sperm cells, and more than 200 other main kinds of cells are among the beautifully and carefully structured cells in your body. There are several ways you may support these cells as they work together to maintain one another's health and the overall functionality of your body. Let's first examine a little bit about cells and their function so that we can fully appreciate how crucial it is to support their work, particularly the activity of the strong and magnificent mitochondria before we discover how to keep them alive and flourishing as long as possible.

Our cells' digesting system is called mitochondria. They take in nutrients, digest them with the help of enzymes and oxygen, and then produce energy that each component may utilize to carry out its specific function. Adenosine triphosphate (ATP), an energy transfer molecule, is produced during this energy production process, also known as "cellular respiration." When a cell needs energy, the mitochondria turn fat or carbohydrates (in the form of glycogen) into energy, which is subsequently transported by ATP to the specific area of the cell that requires it. Almost everybody's process that needs energy receives it via ATP.

Our body's supply of ATP is essentially constant, but it functions like a battery in that we use it up and then, with the aid of our mitochondria, refill it. One of the earliest components of the cell is the mitochondria. They could have started off as single-celled, free-living creatures. They even contain a little bit of DNA of their own that, like the DNA in the cell's nucleus, is susceptible to the effects of our lifestyle choices.

We speak to our mitochondria directly with every movement we make. The mitochondria are turned "on" by movement; conversely, a sedentary lifestyle puts them "off." We really produce more mitochondria when we move our muscles or exercise, which increases the amount of energy we can burn. However, when we let our muscles deteriorate, we have fewer mitochondria, which means we have less energy and fewer calorie-burning furnaces to maintain our weight. Because their mitochondria are primed and ready, fit people often have a lot of energy. Fewer fit persons, on the other hand, have a reduced quantity of mitochondria, just enough to meet their minimal physical demands.

As a consequence, individuals could struggle to do simple chores like getting out of a chair, going up and down stairs, or even getting out of bed. The only thing that separates strong individuals from weaker people, in reality, is what they ask of their muscles. Because muscles are by nature powerful and can be developed stronger with minimal time or work, everyone can have strong muscles. Our bodies want movement.

Our bodies are built to be full of powerful, calorie-burning muscles in their natural form. All of our physical motions, whether conscious or unconscious, are controlled by muscles. We have additional muscles that operate continuously and over which we have no control, in addition to the skeletal muscles that we can actively control, such as our arm, leg, and back muscles. The cardiac muscle, sometimes known as the "heart" muscle, as well as the smooth muscles of our blood vessels, bladder, and digestive system make up this group of uncontrollable muscles.

Every day of our lives, these muscles work continuously to accomplish vital functions including keeping a regular pulse and managing our breathing. Every muscle in the body needs mitochondria to continue functioning, even when we are not exercising. The whole body thus needs energy to carry out these daily tasks, supporting all the systems of the body, such as the neurological system, digestive system, and skeletal system, in addition to the calories our muscles need during exercise.

We need a certain number of calories only to maintain the health of the billions of mitochondria in each of our body's cells. The calorie-burning, energy-producing factories are already at work when we wake up, and regular exercise may encourage these furnaces to burn even more calories. Do you need a little more encouragement to persist with your fitness regimen? I prefer to think of my mitochondria as calorie-burning factories, and the mere fact that my muscles contain 95% of these "factories" inspires me to move more.

Alternatively, I see my mitochondria as the fire under the cauldron of my metabolism, and each step I take adds a piece of wood to the fire, which is "cooking" away my extra pounds and keeping me in shape. Every time we choose to walk rather than drive to the corner store, use the stairs instead of the elevator, or park farther from a mall or shopping center's entrance rather than closer to it, we continue to produce more and more mitochondria.

When you push the vacuum to clean your own home or drag your own baggage through the airport, try to keep your mitochondria in mind. The strength of your energy-producing mitochondria is concentrated by each and every one of these possibilities. Your mitochondria will be more active and fired up if you move more often since you will be using more energy from them. Regularly climbing and descending stairs puts a strain on your mitochondria, which must continually give you a lot of energy.

If you do this often enough, your muscle cells will produce more mitochondria as a kind of compensation, making daily actions simple and uncomplicated. Running up and down stairs will not likely make someone feel the least bit fatigued if they routinely push their bodies. However, someone whose body is unused to the stresses of daily exercise, who seldom sprints up and down stairs, will have fewer mitochondria producing energy and will consequently find this effort to be quite taxing.

Any strong exertion quickly depletes a person's limited supply of mitochondria when they don't regularly exercise, zapping their vitality and leaving their muscles aching and exhausted. They feel winded because their weakened lungs are deficient in oxygen. Their deconditioned heart may be beating and feel overworked. They can even be perspiring from the exertion. They may discover that they were utterly spent and unable to continue exercising or engaging in physical activity until the cells were regenerated, which might take several minutes.

However, if these individuals continued to run up and down stairs every day for a few days, their mitochondria would increase, their muscles would get stronger, and they would quickly discover the exercise to be much simpler to do. The human body is very tough. We are built to be powerful and capable of doing tasks like running up stairs effortlessly. Because of this, your muscles cheerfully and enthusiastically grow with very little work and time, swiftly turning an activity that was formerly difficult into a piece of cake.

The advantages of mitochondria for generating energy are clear and apparent. But the capacity of mitochondria to accelerate weight reduction is also a big benefit for many individuals who have battled with reducing calories and portions to lose weight.

Mitochondria and our weight

I often imagine my body as a house furnace to describe the connection between mitochondria and weight reduction. Imagine if I made the decision to take it easy and not turn on my mitochondrial furnace. The tank would continue to be full while the furnace sat there doing nothing and without using any of my stored calories. The tank would fill up and run out of space if I kept ordering more gasoline.

The fuel oil business would have to leave the excess gasoline in storage tanks near my residence in order to finish the delivery. I'd have to switch on my mitochondrial furnace and burn the extra fuel, as well as embark on a fuel "diet" and minimize my future purchases from the firm to make sure that I only buy as much fuel as I need and nothing more, in order to eliminate this wasteful surplus around my house (and around my hips!).

We don't need more gasoline tanks hanging around our waists. We do need to maintain a healthy balance, work to burn the food we eat, and avoid eating more than we can digest. But more than that, we need a furnace that is always blazing, using those calories. It would be very hard to exercise sufficiently to maintain a healthy weight if burning calories during exercise were the sole benefit of exercise for weight management.

Consider the following scenario to get a sense of how challenging it would be to burn calories just via exercise: Take a 150-pound individual who runs for 30 minutes at a speed of 10 mph; she will burn around 600 calories. She would not be able to burn off all the calories from even that tiny dinner if she had an 8-ounce steak (about 500 calories) and a 7-ounce baked potato (about 250 calories).

To burn away her typical daily calorie intake of thousands of calories sometimes almost two hours a day, she would need to run much longer in a single day. It is obvious that trying to burn off more calories by exercising will not be successful since you will be fighting an uphill battle. You must exercise restraint when it comes to intake and control portion sizes if you want to maintain a stable weight. You can't work out your way out of a poor diet, as the adage goes.

However, burning calories while exercising does play a significant part in weight reduction. Preventing cellular atrophy or death is the main function of exercise in weight reduction. The onset of the inexplicable weight gain that we often attribute to the "age-related" slowdown of the metabolism is mitochondrial loss beyond the age of 40. However, this metabolic slowing has more to do with inactivity and a persistent unwillingness to adopt new behaviors than it does with age!

We often consume the same quantities of food throughout our lives. However, two things happen when you reach old age without engaging in regular exercise or reducing your calorie intake: Your muscle cells shrink or die from lack of usage, leaving you with fewer mitochondria than you had when you were younger. Your capacity to burn mitochondria is also significantly altered. The end result is an unwelcome weight gain that gets worse every year. Fighting a sluggish metabolism doesn't have to leave you feeling hopeless.

The secret to managing your weight and enabling yourself to live a long, healthy life is to have a thorough understanding of the connection between cells, mitochondria, and regular exercise. Let's look more closely at how our bodies age and how we can influence the main factors that slow down, halt, or even reverse metabolic slowdown and physical aging.

CHAPTER 3
WHY DO I FEEL SO OLD?

A lot of individuals fear reaching 40. The unpleasant fact is that if you take care of yourself, there is nothing to worry about, but if you don't, two things start to happen about this time: atrophy and cell death. These natural processes are not unavoidable; there are techniques to combat them, and they are not at all challenging. To understand how to halt this process and turn back the clock, you just need to study what is occurring within your cells.

Life span of a cell

With the combination of a sperm and an egg, we begin life as cells. Cells quickly multiply to produce our bones, hearts, eyes, skin, and every other component of our bodies. This frenzied cell division carries us through the many phases of development, from fetal to baby to toddler to teenager and, eventually, to a mature adult. It involves all of those billions of muscle, brain, nerve, and blood cells. Of course, cells don't merely appear during this period and continue to exist forever. In a continual state of cell turnover, new cells are formed and old cells pass away. Apoptosis, or planned cell death, is preprogrammed in cells, and they wait for a signal from either within or outside the cell to start their own demise.

Apoptosis, which functions as a sculptor's knife to carve out our distinctive characteristics like our fingers and toes, is the body's method of creating itself in accordance with our genetic blueprint while we are still in the process of development. Apoptosis also facilitates memory retention and learning by clearing the brain of unneeded neurons and other debris. Between the ages of 8 and 14, we lose 30 to 40 billion cells daily while still continuously producing new ones.

When we reach maturity and the end of our growing process, a new process of repair and replacement starts. To maintain homeostasis and balance out the formation of new cells, apoptosis speeds up the process and kills 50 billion to 70 billion of our cells every day. Our cells have split so many times by the time we reach the next stage of life around age 40 that the repair and replacement process becomes a bit cumbersome. This process lasts for roughly 20 years.

Our telomeres, the protective caps at the ends of our 46 chromosomes, are snipped off by cells every time they split as they replicate their DNA. The telomeres are almost gone after around 50 divisions, and they provide a strong command to the body to halt cell division. When the DNA is harmed by harmful radiation or chemicals, the cell responds by basically sending out an emergency message. At that point, we leave the stage of repair and replacement and go into the stage of "cell death," also known as "cellular senescence" (from the Latin senex, meaning old age or old man).

Every living organism has a similar life cycle that includes periods of development and maturation, stability, and then a gradual phase of breakdown and decay. Every living thing, whether it be a plant, an animal, or a person, goes through a natural cycle of life and death. However, there are certain things we can do to speed this process, slow it down, or maybe even reverse it, much as the nature of our gardener's caring can either help her flowers enjoy a lengthy flowering time or wilt prematurely. Scientists have been debating numerous hypotheses of how aging affects the body for decades.

Some people think that accumulated oxidation is the main cause of harm to our cells. When our cells lose electrons due to oxidation, which takes place when free radicals are created by cellular respiration or ingested from environmental exposure to things like secondhand smoke, pesticides, and toxins, oxidation takes place. Just consider what happens to iron when it is oxidized; it rusts. The outcome is devastating.

According to this theory, the apoptosis mechanism might malfunction if enough chemicals in our cells, including our DNA, are destroyed. Our body reaches a tipping point at that time, our tissues and organs begin to disintegrate, and illness begins to spread. Recently, researchers have focused their attention on this same mechanism occurring inside the mitochondrial DNA. Many believe that understanding how our mitochondria work as we age will help us solve the enigma of aging and that the way aging impacts our health depends on the quantity and health of our mitochondria.

The two ideas of aging may be related, according to a newer line of study that contends that our mitochondria really communicate with our cells' telomeres to determine whether they should shorten and speed up aging or not, which would aid to slow down or halt the aging process. I anticipate that over the next years, as science continues to advance, we will learn even more important things about how the human body ages. But for the time being, it would seem to be best for us to get to know and care for these really important small power plants.

What can we do to ensure that we have a sufficient number of healthy mitochondria to instruct our telomeres to remain long indefinitely? Our genes do contribute to this, but not in the most significant way. Perhaps your parents and grandparents have lived a long life. Nevertheless, don't count on living a long life by yourself. Only 30% of our lifetime, according to experts, is controlled by our DNA. We are unable to replace inherited genes that increase our risk of developing cancer or heart disease.

However, we may take precautions to shield ourselves from the worst of those genetic signals. According to the emerging area of "epigenetics," which investigates everything that occurs to your genes after birth, certain actions turn on good genes and turn off negative ones, or vice versa. The amount of "load" on our bodies is a function of the decisions we make throughout our lives.

Our genetic load and risk of genetic damage decrease as we make more healthy decisions. (The phrase "Our genes load the pistol, but our environment pulls the trigger" is one of the epigenetics axioms.) Even if we lead "clean" lifestyles, we all live in a contemporary, sometimes hazardous world where we constantly face environmental threats to the integrity of our DNA.

Each person's genome sustains damage over time, and every time a cell splits and copies its DNA, the chance of mutation rises. By managing the environment in which those genes are expressed and protecting our cells from environmental threats like stress, poor nutrition, chemicals, insufficient sleep, and a host of other elements that cause oxidative stress and have been shown to harm our genes, we can have the greatest influence on how those genes are expressed.

However, we have a highly effective attack on our side as well as a defense in the form of eccentric exercise. Animal studies have shown that eccentric exercise, the kind that the ESSENTRICS approach emphasizes, interacts directly with the mitochondria in human cells to lower oxidative stress on a molecular level, so directly battles aging. Another special substance found in our bodies, telomerase, enhances mitochondrial activity to prevent those signals that might otherwise shorten our telomeres.

And what has been shown to boost telomerase, preserve telomeres, limit cell death, prevent mitochondrial loss and all benefits that may help us live longer and have better quality of life as we age? Exercise. Have you noticed any changes in your body recently, such as a decrease in energy, an unexplained weight increase, bad posture, or a change in your body shape? The signals that your DNA and cells have been receiving for years are reflected in these modifications.

But the decisions you make each day, beginning now, may stop these signals and delay the events that lead to cell death. Take action right now to start Looking Younger. We scarcely see the progression of our life cycle on a daily basis since changes take place one cell at a time at the cellular level. Only in hindsight, when we contrast how our lives formerly were with how they are now, do we realize it. Children are more likely to come to this knowledge when they suddenly have the ability to do tasks they had previously been unable to perform, such as riding a bike, reaching into high cabinets for cookies, or participating in certain sports.

These achievements serve as concrete markers that help a youngster recognize his or her own development and maturing. On the other hand, the things we can no longer perform become the milestones we notice when we enter the window of change following repair and replacement. We may no longer be able to play particular sports, or we could find it harder to sprint to catch a bus.

Or, we could even discover that activities we once took for granted, like cracking jar lids or lugging heavy goods inside the vehicle, now present a challenge. When tasks we completed easily last summer, like mowing the lawn or gardening for hours, have turned into a tiresome effort this summer, we become aware of changes in our energy levels. The most startling discovery can occur when last year's clothing no longer fit. We seldom perceive this process since it moves along so slowly. We only notice it when we compare images of ourselves taken over the years and note how our form and weight have changed along with the appearance of new wrinkles.

Thankfully, we are blissfully oblivious to the fact that we are steadily deteriorating due to cell death on a regular basis. Who wants a daily reminder of aging? But we get nothing from this gradual fading. Those sobering insights might sometimes be just what we need to remain watchful and stop premature aging. So that we can develop the awareness that will motivate us to take action, let's take a deeper look at what is happening here, at the cellular level.

The message to not repair or replace dead cells grows increasingly aggressive at the age of 40, and with each decade that follows. That message is feeble while we are in our early forties, but it soon picks up steam. Other physical systems are also degrading similar to the cellular decline. Both men's and women's testosterone and estrogen levels fall. Our hearts and lungs deteriorate, particularly if we don't exercise much. Our equilibrium deteriorates. Increased calcification in our blood arteries limits the free flow of blood throughout the body.

The cumulative impact of any of these unfavorable changes might be rather significant. The majority of us have seen family members, friends, and grandparents age and are shocked by their quick decline in their seventies or eighties, or even earlier, but going through it oneself is a different story. Despite the fact that medical science has advanced significantly over the last several decades, scientists have not yet clearly linked all the dots, and they continue to be unsure of the best ways to maintain youth and stop cell aging.

When I first began considering cells as the building blocks of life and development, I was particularly curious about two things:
1. What causes cells to be maintained?
2. Why does this period of maintenance come to an end? I was very interested in finding out whether we might postpone or even stop the

communication that triggers cell death in order to extend the repair and replacement phase.

We can infer a person's age just by looking at their posture or level of energy among a group of adults who were picked at random. Compared to 60 or 70-year-olds, people in their twenties often have more energy, are stronger, and stand up straighter. The physical contrasts between a young adult and an elderly one are striking. What has changed to bring about these visible indicators of aging? As we've mentioned, the body constantly produces new cells to replace damaged and dead ones, resulting in a continual turnover of cells from the time we are born.

The innate signal to replace and repair damaged and dying cells are sent from infancy through adolescence, but it becomes less strong as we become older. Something fresh must occur to mark a change in order to turn off the maintenance notice. It must be more than simply chronological aging for that "something new" to differ so widely from person to person. We must demonstrate to our body the importance of these cells if we want to maintain the "repair and replace" command rather than letting the "let die" command take control. We are aware that only when muscle cells are not in use do they get the signal to atrophy.

Therefore, it follows that the best method to stop the process of cell death is to declare loudly, "I still need these muscles! They're still in use by me! And the only way to achieve so is to utilize each and every one of your 620 muscles every single day in order to stop any message of atrophy from reaching any portion of your body. You may have instinctively known this all along if you are used to routine exercise: As long as you are utilizing a muscle, its cells will continue to be healed and replaced. In the fields of medicine, surgery, and physiotherapy, we see this knowledge in action.

For instance, hospital patients are urged to get out of bed and start exercising as soon as the doctor gives the all-clear, which is sometimes only hours following surgery. Even if getting up may feel excruciating to the patient, physicians are aware of the negative effects of being inactive after surgery. The goal of exercise after surgery is to avoid muscular atrophy and shrinkage, which would make complete recovery considerably more difficult and unsuccessful.

When you begin in a condition of reasonably excellent health, and particularly robust health, this idea is much more persuasive. In 2011, research on muscular atrophy and chronological aging was carried out at the University of Pittsburgh. 40 elite recreational athletes between the ages of 40 and 81 who exercised four or five times a week had their muscle tissue cross-sectioned by the researchers.

Astonishing findings were made by the researchers after examining the subjects' quadriceps strength, body composition, and an MRI of their quadriceps: A 74-year-old triathlete's lean muscle mass was about equivalent to that of a 40-year-old who worked out on a regular basis. The research refuted previously held beliefs and "common knowledge" that aging naturally caused a loss in muscular mass and strength. Instead, the researchers received unambiguous evidence that the cause of muscle cell loss was inactivity rather than aging. These results apply to non-athletes as well as athletes. According to statistics, the ordinary individual who leads a slightly sedentary, somewhat active lifestyle and engages in a minimal level of daily exercise loses 7 to 8 percent of her body's cells on average every ten years.

On the other hand, an active individual who regularly exercises while utilizing all of her muscles loses just 2 to 3 percent of their cells on average every ten years. By age 60, the more sedentary individual will have lost up to 25% of her muscle cells, compared with an average of 8% loss in the active person. This is such a significant improvement. Given that eccentric exercise is the most effective and efficient kind of muscle training, ESSENTRICS can assist you in achieving these outcomes more quickly than any other program.

After completing an 8-week program to compare the effects of concentric versus eccentric training, a Swiss study of heart disease patients between the ages of 40 and 66 found that, despite experiencing a similar level of exertion, those who had followed the eccentric program were able to produce four times as much power as those who had followed the concentric program.

In other words, the eccentric exercisers received four times the benefit for the same amount of exertion. Significantly, neither their blood pressure nor any other cardiac stress indicators increased at all. This suggests a less risky kind of exercise for those with heart conditions while they recover from a potentially fatal cardiac attack. For the rest of us, it simply means that we may develop our strength, flexibility, leanness, and youthful appearance without having to spend hours on the treadmill or potentially even break a sweat!

CHAPTER 4
FITNESS AND DISEASE PREVENTION

Another aging myth that many naively believe is that we'll all become sick at some time and that illness and aging go hand in hand. It's untrue. You may prevent the start of illness through a variety of dietary and lifestyle choices, but one of the most effective is exercise's capacity to increase muscle mass. Fitness may prevent sickness as well as help you lose weight and have more energy. We'll examine how the circulatory, digestive, and neurological systems of your body are impacted by your muscular strength.

These may deteriorate with age, but not if you make a commitment to exercise. The body is comparable to a multi-system complicated automobile that must have all of its systems functioning properly for the vehicle to be able to move. The wheels, engine, transmission, and brakes are analogous to the muscles, the neurological system, the cardiovascular system, and the digestive system, respectively. The automobile won't move if any of those components are malfunctioning. The automobile could still operate, but it will probably run poorly if the components are rusty and worn out. Healthy, strong, and flexible muscles may help in this situation.

The muscles have a variety of functions, including maintaining system health, helping the digestive system remove waste materials, helping the circulatory system distribute blood to all of the body's cells, and much more. The systems quickly grow worn out and breakdown if strong, healthy muscles aren't performing in unison with them. This makes us feel and seem unwell, makes us more prone to illness, and makes us recover from illnesses more slowly than is required.

Your health is maintained by having strong, flexible muscles, which also aid in your quick and complete recovery from illness. The muscular system is the most crucial system in your body if you want to stay youthful and healthy. All of the other systems that keep you alive are immediately impacted when you let your muscular system deteriorate. All other systems will age quickly due to misuse and deterioration if there aren't strong, flexible muscles. One Danish research examined the effects of heavy alcohol intake, smoking, inactivity, and obesity on anticipated lifespan.

Data on illness prevalence and life tables from the Danish Health Interview Survey's more than 14,000 individuals were pooled by the researchers. They discovered that, on average, those who are physically inactive would live 5 to 8 years less than those who are physically active. We are aware that 620 muscles will atrophy if they are not used. When this occurs, it will be harder for us to maintain our health since the body's systems that keep us healthy will start to deteriorate due to atrophy.

Cardiovascular system

Our most vital muscle has to be protected at all costs since it is the heart. In order to maintain the cardiovascular system healthy and operating to its best potential, the muscular system is crucial. In order to increase circulation and lessen part of our cardiovascular burden, the muscular system is built to cooperate with the heart, veins, and arteries. Reducing the burden on the heart protects vital components of the cardiovascular system from damage that might lead to inflammation and heart disease.

Our bodies' ability to efficiently circulate blood has a direct influence on muscle function. Active muscles are made to act as pumps, promoting blood flow. The vessels, which normally would have to conduct all the pumping and transportation of blood alone, are relieved of part of the burden by the muscles' pumping motion. The vessels can't pump as efficiently on their own as they can when the muscles are working alongside them.

This implies that certain cells are not getting blood rich with nutrients and oxygen, making us more susceptible to disease and chronic fatigue. The sensation that we are dragging all day and can never catch up on sleep. Sounds recognizable? To keep us youthful, we need muscles that are working and supplying nutrition and eliminating waste. The circulatory system, or as I sometimes say, "from the brain to brawn," is the mechanism that transports blood throughout the whole body. Every cell in the body receives nutrient-rich, oxygen-rich blood from the circulatory system, which also serves as a trash collection system by removing waste materials like toxins and dead cells on the way back.

Our cells won't get vital nutrients from a sluggish circulatory system, and harmful pollutants won't be removed from our bodies. We are left feeling and appearing worn out as a result: dull, lifeless skin is a telltale sign of a slow circulatory system. According to a recent study, the New York Times revealed that exercising has other benefits outside of just washing our skin. The exploratory study from McMaster University in Ontario tracked a group of inactive men and women over 65 to examine the impact their exercise habits had on their skin. It was presented in 2014 at the annual conference of the American Medical Society for Sports Medicine.

For three months, the researchers had this previously inactive group exercise hard (at 65 percent of the patients' maximal heart rates) for 30 minutes twice a week. The skin of the participants had undergone significant alteration, and it now more closely matched that of persons in their twenties, the researchers found after examining skin samples from the subjects. Myokines, a kind of protein produced by the muscle, are thought to be released in response to exercise; these myokines travel from the muscle into the circulation and induce changes in cells far from the cells from which they were released.

According to the skin samples, myokine levels increased by 50% after the commencement of the trial. Genetic changes were occurring in exercisers, and these genetic alterations were showing up as younger, dewier, less-lined skin. Nothing can match the vitality that healthy circulation offers to the skin in terms of face creams. Full-body circulation is more effective in cleansing and nourishing the skin than massages or facials. I like my lotions, facials, and massages, but nothing can make your skin shine like a good full-body exercise!

We just need to engage in 10 minutes of vigorous activity each day to enhance blood flow, eliminate toxins, and provide the body with nutrients and oxygen that will give it vitality. Nothing drains us more than spending the whole day inactive. That is true of everybody who works in an office. And nothing brightens our eyes like a few minutes of physical activity. Large full-body motions, such as those used in Classical Stretch, ESSENTRICS, and tai chi, all engage the cardiovascular system's muscles and promote blood circulation without putting any strain on the joints.

They are a great substitute for conventional cardio exercises on the market. We have greater energy when the circulatory system is working properly. We think more clearly as a result of our brains receiving more oxygen. Simply put, we feel better overall. Numerous research on the health advantages of tai chi has been conducted by the Harvard School of Medicine. It's interesting to note that Chinese people have practiced tai chi for generations and that many of them have lived most of their lives without experiencing any exercise-related ailments.

People still practice tai chi in parks, workplaces, and other public spaces across China. Because they regularly practice tai chi, the Chinese are renowned for their longevity and excellent health. Additionally, tai chi-like movements are beneficial in preventing coronary artery disease and had an impact on a number of factors associated with the disease, such as lowered blood pressure, an increase in exercise capacity, and improved cholesterol levels. This was demonstrated by studies like those on tai chi conducted by the Harvard Medical School.

This result has significant ramifications, particularly in light of the fact that coronary artery disease is the main cause of mortality in America. These exercise regimens ease the stress on the arteries brought on by a buildup of plaque in arterial walls with their broad, sweeping muscular motions. Muscle contraction and relaxation result in a pumping motion that helps the blood circulate into the extremities and back to the heart. Large muscular contractions assist the heart muscle in pumping blood, relieving the strain on the organ and spreading the work of complete circulation.

Taiji has been shown to lower participants' systolic blood pressure by up to 22 points and their diastolic blood pressure by up to 12 points, according to an assessment of the subject's ability to prevent chronic heart disease for the Cochrane Database Systemic Reviews. LDL-C, triglycerides, and total cholesterol were all reduced in two investigations. Taiji, a traditional Chinese exercise, and other comparable practices like ESSENTRICs have a strong cardiovascular foundation.

I've looked for alternatives since I personally don't like doing standard cardio exercises like aerobics or jogging on a treadmill. Don't stop doing them if you love them, but long-term use of these high-impact exercises has been shown to harm joints. Many of my customers are avid runners who want to keep running for the rest of their lives. You merely need to safeguard your joints with the right strengthening and concomitant stretching activities, and you ought to be able to achieve that. Sadly, hardly many runners take the effort to safeguard their joints.

I've dealt with a lot of runners over 45 who had to quit running due to injury or discomfort in their joints. Nobody should be forced to give up their beloved activity, particularly if it benefits the cardiovascular system or other bodily systems. However, players must take preventative measures to ensure that their joints endure a lifetime.

Digestive system

The purpose of the digestive system is to break down the food we consume into molecules that can pass past the walls of our cells and be used as fuel by our mitochondria, the cellular furnaces that burn calories. An intricate network of chemical processing stations and tubes (the esophagus and intestines) facilitates digestion (liver, pancreas, kidneys, and bladder). The system begins in the mouth and is completed when the waste products are out, excess fat is transferred to fat storage units, and nutrients are supplied to the cells. When everything is working properly, we should be completely unconscious that this astounding achievement is being performed within the body's borders. As the meal moves through the system, we shouldn't experience any pain, discomfort, or bloating.

The torso is where the digestive system is located. Every individual has enough room at birth for the digestive system to operate effectively. The caveat is that we only have adequate room when we are standing or sitting upright and when our spine is at its longest. Poor posture shortens the space needed to accommodate the digestive system properly and crushes the spine. As a consequence, the tubes and organs are crushed and forced outward against the body's walls. By constricting their area, you cannot expect the factories and pipelines to operate without a hitch. The flow of the meal is made unpleasant, ineffective, and painful by this restriction of space. It doesn't need a scientific investigation to demonstrate to us how common stomach pain is among Americans.

A pharmacy's aisles are lined with rows upon rows of over-the-counter digestive drugs, which may be seen by anybody who enters. Exercise may benefit two digestive system components:

1. The upper section, where issues like acid reflux, coughing, and heartburn may happen.

2. The lower region, where problems including poor elimination and constipation are frequent.

Poor posture mostly affects the upper portion of the body, or the region of the body from the waist up, since it causes the spine to sag forward, crushing the rib cage and shortening our height. The rib cage must go someplace as the body sags forward, which is how the esophageal tubing becomes clogged. The lungs, esophagus, heart, and liver are all jammed within and competing with one another for room by pushing against one another since the only direction the ribs can go is backward toward your spine. The food you just ate is attempting to enter your stomach while everything else is crammed into the space around your rib cage. Simply adjusting your posture can make digestion more pleasant and simpler. All of the torso's muscles must be lengthened and strengthened to attain good posture.

The intestinal portion of the digestive system, which most people mistakenly refer to as the stomach, is the second component that needs strong muscles. When we feel bloated, it is most likely not our stomach at all but rather our intestines. Between the waist and the rectum, the intestines form a 30-foot-long hose or tube. The lining of the intestines has a particular sort of muscle that unconsciously pushes the excrement through without our awareness.

The feces wouldn't be able to pass through the intestines without these unconscious muscles. The abdominal muscles are made to cooperate with the intestinal muscles in pushing feces through the intestines, much like other "in-groups" of muscles that serve as assistants to specific groups of muscles. Our abdominal muscles will be weak if we lead a sedentary lifestyle.

Because the intestinal muscles won't have anything to push against, the flow of feces through our intestines will be slowed down, which will cause the feces to harden and cause constipation. We refer to persons with enormous projecting abdomens as having "giant stomachs," but in reality, these people really have weak abdominal muscles, which is why their intestines are protruding! Again, the intestines dangle when the abdominal muscles are weak because nothing is holding them in.

The "toothpaste effect" comes to mind: The toothpaste comes out more easily the more we twist and press the toothpaste tube. Since our intestines are tubes, they need all the assistance we can muster in order to facilitate quick and painless disposal. The "innards" become more pliable with relaxed, easy motions that entail twisting and turning and as much torso movement as is safe. This facilitates simple evacuation.

CHAPTER 5
HOW TO WORKOUT

Many of us want to seem 10 years younger and 10 years lighter than we already do. To succeed, we need muscles that are both strong and flexible and excellent posture. Any atrophy that may be leaving us feeling flimsy, rigid, or low on energy is something we want to reverse. Through a series of stretching and strengthening exercises, we must first stop the atrophy. Because I have seen such incredible outcomes in everyone who has ever committed to performing ESSENTRICS for 30 minutes a day, I'm thrilled to share these routines with you.

You've seen the studies; you are aware that eccentric exercise is the most secure, effective, and potent way to stretch and strengthen. You are aware that your body will become more flexible and balanced, and you won't sustain any injuries. With longer, slimmer muscles and a much larger concentration of energy-producing, fat-burning mitochondria powering your cells, you know you can get the "dancer's body" you've always desired. You'll convince your DNA that you're alive and that every single cell in your body is necessary, which will activate every muscle in your body and stop the aging process.

No early cell death for you! Your journey to looking younger is underway. Start these workouts slowly and don't push yourself too hard. Do the exercises for 30 minutes each day for the first week or two, being careful to move slowly and unwind as you go. Actually, if you don't strive to build your muscles, you will strengthen more quickly. You'll advance far more quickly if you maintain your calm than if you overextend yourself, lose motivation, and give up.

You could ask whether these activities might strengthen you if you are in excellent form. Do you recall the tale of Anik, the wounded ballet dancer who, after two weeks of practicing ESSENTRICS, recovered even more powerfully? Try it! The outcomes will be self-evident. Any workout will be more challenging if you are weak, out of shape, or atrophying to any degree. But please try not to give up. You'll experience a heavy weight on your arms. You could discover that even slightly straightening your back can cause you to tremble and perspire excessively.

Don't attempt harder than 20 to 30 minutes every day. According to my experience, these workouts will start to become simpler and you'll stop sweating after two weeks. Regardless of how awful our physical condition may be, I am always amazed by how robust the human body is and how eager it is to be revived when given a chance. These ESSENTRICS exercises are intended to be performed daily for around 30 minutes. A half-hour of daily exercise that doesn't injure you or turn you into a fitness fanatic has positive effects on the human body.

30 minutes of these full-body stretches and strengthening exercises is all you need to keep in shape. Like doing too little, doing too much may lead to a host of issues. The crucial factor is constancy. Exercises should be stopped right once

if they cause a sudden, "knifelike" discomfort. Knife-like pain is a warning sign that your body cannot do the workouts properly; continuing might result in harm. If you just find them demanding and exhausting, keep continuing; that is what they are meant to be. Keep track of how fast your body adapts to the difficulties as you do various routines.

Be amazed by the human body's remarkable receptivity to stimuli and how it adjusts itself effectively and swiftly whenever new demands and strains are put on it. Miraculous! Your muscles will react quickly to strength and flexibility training, even if you have never worked out before or have let your body become inactively inert. The advantages of this training will also motivate you to keep moving forward and taking on more difficult tasks.

The ideal time to work out? Every time you say you will! Find the time of day when you like working out the most and are least likely to skip a workout by working with your biorhythms. Building a persistent exercise routine will be much easier if you workout first thing in the morning. After all, if you prioritize your exercises, the rest of your life won't have a chance to interfere with them. However, if noon or an hour before bed works better for you, go with it. Just make sure you get in your daily 30 minutes. Do it for your brain, heart, muscles, and cells! A University of Copenhagen research found that even one session of vigorous exercise may enhance long-term memory.

However, consistency is key, and those tremendous brain advantages can fade if you stop working out. Have fun doing them, that's the most essential thing. Your body will feel so amazing after using them that you won't think it's possible to exercise. Forget the adage "no pain, no gain"; your body already knows what's best. Your body will be grateful to you for making it feel so rejuvenated, at ease, and full of oxygen.

Straighten your posture

In addition to making you seem confident and young, good posture lifts your spine higher, creating room for all of your organs to operate properly in the location that "God" intended for them. Poor posture reduces the room for your organs while giving you rounded shoulders and a bent spine that makes you seem exhausted and aged. The organs squish outward because they are forced lower by the spine's shrinkage and have nowhere else to go. We seem fatter than we really are as a result of this.

Therefore, having excellent posture helps us seem younger and slimmer, but having poor posture makes us appear older and heavier. However, if your muscles are weak or exhibit any degree of atrophy, it may be difficult to improve your posture and straighten your back. Having excellent posture is simple, natural, and pleasant when our muscles are strong and flexible. Additionally, maintaining a straight posture for prolonged periods of time is simpler and more pleasant when muscles are strong and flexible.

The only way to maintain the spine in excellent shape for the rest of your life is to exercise it. In particular, if we spend more than 8 hours a day sitting at a computer and the remaining time on a couch in front of the TV, movement is crucial to preserving healthy posture. If having a nice appearance isn't incentive enough, think about how important correct posture is for maintaining optimal organ function. The cardiovascular, neurological, digestive, and skeletal systems of the body are all adversely impacted by poor posture.

Poor posture prevents our lungs from taking in enough oxygen, which causes oxygen deprivation in the brain and muscles and leaves us feeling perpetually fatigued and lethargic. Additionally, poor posture strains the digestive system, which may result in constipation, bloating, cramps, heartburn, gas, and cramp-like symptoms. The circulatory system's ability to circulate blood that provides energy is compromised by poor posture. Sedentary behavior often leads to poor posture.

The hundreds of muscles needed to keep the spine upright deteriorate due to inactivity, which also starts the process of accelerated aging. The spine cannot be held in an upright posture for more than a few minutes until weak, atrophied muscles tire and collapse. If your muscles are weak, it will be difficult, if not impossible, to maintain an appropriate posture. Don't give up, however; our muscles are only waiting for us to build them up. All it takes is a little daily workout, and in just a few short weeks, we should have beautiful posture. The muscles that the body has that were created by God are powerful and long-lasting.

They are not made to be fragile! With a little effort, they may quickly get stronger. 33 tiny wedge-shaped bones, known as vertebrae, make up the spine, which curves gently in a double-S pattern from the base of the head to the tailbone. The double-S curvature offers the spine flexibility, allowing it to compress and extend like an accordion. The spine lengthens as we draw it upward, making us seem taller; conversely, when we let the spine compress, we appear shorter.

If we were to be measured in each of our many postural postures, we would truly be either taller or shorter. Numerous muscles in the torso may be used to support proper posture. These muscles, which extend from the spine to our shoulders, ribs, cranium, legs, and hips, vary in size from tiny to enormous. Together, they help to maintain the spine's strength, flexibility, and proper alignment. Each and every one of these muscles is essential to maintaining proper posture, and each one has to be equally strong and stretched in order for the spine to stay in equilibrium.

When the muscles in our spine are balanced, we enjoy a relaxed, ideal posture. Exercises are necessary to maintain the spinal muscles' ability to move in all directions since the spine is designed to move in every way conceivable. Exercising all the muscles necessary for excellent posture could seem like an overwhelming task, but I'll show you that it's really pretty easy. Only your own devotion to your body is challenging. Are you prepared to do these workouts for the rest of your life at least three times each week? I've put up a sample of exercises that will increase your flexibility and strength in all the muscles necessary for healthy posture.

Additionally, these workouts might help you manage your weight and offer you a more beautiful form by toning your torso.

Most likely, your mother told you to "stand up straight!" Though sometimes we're not entirely sure what "straight" implies, she was right. The mistaken idea that overstrengthening the shoulder, arm, and upper back muscles can promote excellent posture, fitness and sports training often do so. A strong, stiff, immobile back and a strong, straight, completely movable back, however, vary greatly from one another. For strengthening to be safe and effective and prevent premature atrophy, it must be counterbalanced with an equivalent amount of dynamic flexibility.

Anyone participating in a sport or fitness activity should take a step back and evaluate the outcomes. Consider if your action creates more issues than it resolves. Admitting that the training we have grown to love could be hurting us is quite challenging. It is difficult to acknowledge that a trainer we admire and who has likely grown to be a friend is teaching us exercises that are really hurting us. It might be challenging to stop engaging in fitness activities that are detrimental to you since life is often about decisions and facts.

Considering the fitness sector, being inactive is the worst thing we can do for our posture. Sedentary lifestyles always cause premature aging, permanent atrophy, and bad posture. Our poor posture puts us at risk for cardiovascular, digestive, skeletal, and neurological issues. We shouldn't allow our bodies to hinder our enjoyment of life since it's enjoyable! Life is a strong force that does not give up easily. Every second of life is a battle for survival. However, time advances gradually and slowly.

Despite the passage of time, we must remain watchful and refrain from aging too quickly. I've shown you that, as long as you make a commitment to everyday exercise, you do have a choice. We cannot halt time because it never does. We must choose to stop cell death, atrophy, and bad posture if we want to feel young. A sin of omission, as opposed to commission, is doing nothing. Inaction is a decision to allow your body to deteriorate earlier than necessary. The option to maintain one's vitality, health, and youth is to take action. Our DNA has a hazy expiry date at birth. But the quality of the life we will lead from conception to death is not something we are born with.

Free will and the element of choice have a role in the quality of our lives. I've shown you that we can influence how quickly we approach death. I've shown you how regular exercise may help you keep a healthy posture, plenty of energy, strength, and mobility. You can decide how much chronic weariness and discomfort you will experience or how great you will feel. Your decision to be idle or active is what gives you power.

I've shown you that if you don't exercise regularly, you'll age terribly and quickly. Painful conditions include arthritis, atrophy, and weakness. Action or inactivity are our only two obvious options. There isn't a third option. There is no putting off the decision until you are in the right frame of mind.

Your opportunity to live a vigorous, thrilling, and energizing life far into your golden years is all you are "putting off."

There is no urgency or franticness; time moves at a peaceful and steady pace. We don't have to work out feverishly to stay up with time; 30 minutes of leisurely exercise every day will do the trick. You just need to spend 30 minutes a day if you want to be able to dress and undress without help, have a lively social life with friends and family, and not get tired quickly. You just need to exercise your muscles for 30 minutes a day to maintain them healthy and pain-free. Most of us don't have a lot of demands; all we want is to feel youthful instead of old, healthy instead of unwell.

We must exercise for 30 minutes every day for a minimum of 30 days in order to slow down and reverse the effects of aging. I'm done now! We need to keep our back muscles strong and flexible if we wish to have excellent posture. Without consistent exercise, our muscles are designed to contract and atrophy. If that occurs, we won't have the energy to keep our posture upright. If we don't exercise, calories aren't burnt to offer us energy, and we'll feel weary all the time. If we want energy, we need to fuel the mitochondria to give us energy. After reading this book, you will be aware of the internal processes that cause aging.

You are also aware of how to keep your body from aging. You may now choose. I'm here to inform you of your options and to persuade you to go in the direction of better health. I've made the decision to lead an active lifestyle, and I'm happy with how things are going. Being active doesn't guarantee that I won't become sick; I'm not naïve about that. I've had my fair share of serious diseases and shattered bones, so I understand what they're like.

I know I can survive them and emerge stronger because of that experience. I have a decent chance of recovering quickly since I'm active; the odds are in my favor. Additionally, it implies that I'll stay young and energetic far into my senior years. I can enjoy my life since I'm active. I can enjoy my friends and my kid. I can't wait to go on vacation. I can anticipate a new experience every year, which makes me look forward to it. I've stopped looking forward to reaching "old age." I now understand how to have a pleasant life up to my death.

That's what I'm doing right now. What more could a person want? I was struck by the realization that everyone has the same potent energy of life rushing through their veins as I watched my father fight to survive in his last months. We just need to awaken the energy of life inside us, and it will reply a thousand times over. The mitochondria will activate with the tiniest motions, igniting the flames of life!